The Guide to Getting Help

A handbook for navigating the helping professions

By Ian Felton MA, LPC

For those close to me who've been patient while I flopped around on the earth like a fish out of water.

Cover art by Ian Felton © 2019
Published by jerk cat publishing

Visit the author's website: www.ianfelton.com

ISBN: 978-0-9986909-3-3

Acknowledgments

I want to thank everyone who seeks help, as this act shows bravery, humility, and a desire to make one's life better. Through this act, all of humanity can benefit. Seeking and receiving help is a gift we give ourselves. May we all find the strength and opportunity to receive it.

I want to thank my supervisor, Matthew Paymar, whose similar spirit regarding making finding help easier aided in inspiring this book. I also appreciate his feedback and insights into the field that provided me with a sizable portion of the knowledge I used to write this book.

I also want to thank my friends and colleagues, David Swirnoff and Ryan Peterson, who helped me to develop the organization of the chapters and rethink some finer points in addition to supporting the overall effort.

Lastly, my partner, Jennifer Buege, contributed her fantastic editing skills and tried to keep our cat, Bert, calm so I could work.

Table of Contents

CHAPTER 1
The Quick Guide to Getting Help

Before going a step further, I want to provide a list of quick, simple steps to follow to get help. I don't want you to feel like you need to read an entire book before looking for it. These steps will hopefully guide you down the path to finding the help you want. Getting help the first time can be a scary but rewarding experience. If you're nervous, try to remember that therapists are there to help you and are held to high ethical standards, including keeping everything you discuss confidential (with certain limitations; see Chapter 12).

1. If you don't have a referral to a counselor and you plan on using insurance, find out from your insurance company if you have mental health benefits (or behavioral health benefits). If you do, find out your deductible and co-pay. If you have a co-pay, it's what you'll need to pay for each session once you've

met your deductible. It's very important to do this step first to avoid wasting a lot of time searching for providers only to find out they aren't in your insurance company's network. Tell the person on the phone that you're seeking a list of their in-network behavioral health, or mental health, providers. Then ask whether the insurer has an online search tool. Many insurance companies have a search tool on their websites that you can use to find counselors in your area that are in your insurance company's network.

2.   If you can't find anyone in your insurance company's network, you can still look for providers that will bill your insurance plan as an out-of-network provider. One note: Your deductible may be higher if using an out-of-network-provider. In this case, search the web for something like "counselors" or "psychotherapists." Look at a few therapist profiles and websites in your area and make a small list of phone numbers and email addresses.

3. ***If you don't have insurance and can't afford to see a counselor, don't give up!*** If you don't have internet access at home, go to the local library or somewhere with public internet access. Do a search for "sliding scale psychotherapy" or "free counseling." Many counselors offer some time slots to those who can't afford counseling, and sometimes there's a community counseling center that offers free or reduced-cost services.

4. Now it's time to start contacting therapists. Don't be afraid to reach out to several people at once. Typically, a counselor will follow up within a day or two, sometimes quicker. I know this may seem like a long time. Keep in mind, though, that many practitioners don't have assistants or support staff and they must handle all of their communications themselves. If they're in sessions all day or have the day off, it can take a little time for them to respond. If it's a real emergency, call 911. Otherwise, hang in

there. If you contact three or four counselors, someone will get back to you soon. Don't worry if you feel overwhelmed; it's natural. Be patient with yourself and with this part of the process.

5.   Once you're in contact with someone, they'll either have a short phone call with you or communicate via email if that's how you reached out to them. This part of the process is to get an initial appointment, or intake, scheduled where you may be able to talk with the counselor about what's going on in your life and ask a few questions. Double-check with the counselor regarding what payment is due at the first session and what payment methods they accept. Some counselors don't take credit cards, so you'll want to be certain you come prepared.

6.   Before your first visit, the counselor may ask you to fill out some forms. This is normal. If they don't ask you to do so before your visit, you'll likely fill them out in the waiting room when you arrive for

your first visit. Most of the forms will relate to basic information about yourself, but have your insurance card handy as well. These forms are necessary to set up your file and to gain your consent to begin working with your therapist. There's nothing else you need to do before your first visit. However, if you'd like, feel free to use this time to reflect on what you want to work on in therapy by journaling or just thinking it through.

7.   Now it's the day of your appointment. Make sure you know the directions to your counselor's office as well as where to park. Try to arrive five minutes early (or more if your counselor has requested it) so you don't miss any of your precious session time. Most counselors are on a tight schedule and won't be able to give you extra time at the end if you're late.

8.   Meeting your therapist is many times an exciting moment. You're venturing toward having a better life. It's normal to feel a lot of emotion and perhaps conflicts about sharing feelings and emotions with

someone you just met. Be patient with yourself. Taking this step is brave, no matter who you are. Congratulate yourself on caring enough about yourself to do this.

One other consideration: It's important to determine whether you feel like you can have a trusting relationship with your counselor. Most of the time you will, but if you feel like you don't connect with them after three or four sessions, go back to your list and try the next counselor. It's normal to see a counselor for months or even years, so you want to be able to trust them and feel like you can work with him or her.

CHAPTER 2
Introduction

I wrote this book as a handbook for those seeking help in any area that can be considered mental health. For no good reason, seeking treatment still has stigma attached to it. I want to remove as many barriers as I can for those who want help but are confused or ashamed to ask questions. I'm a mental health professional who's sought help myself, so I'm familiar with both sides of the process. My goal is to answer as many basic questions as I can for those seeking psychotherapy services.

Why get help?

There are far more reasons to get help than not to get it. Nevertheless, for many of us, the reasons we use for not getting help drown out the voice inside of us that really, really would like to ask someone to hear us and to see us. We recognize that there are things going on in our lives that we want to sort out, but we say, "No one wants to hear my problems," "Just suck it up," "Quit being a baby," or any number of other statements that we've picked up along the way that make us believe that our problems aren't worth wasting anyone's time on.

I'm here to tell you that there are many people who would say in response, "I want to hear what's bothering you," or "You don't have to deal with this problem alone," or "There's no shame in coming here; I'm here to help."

There's an endless list of reasons why people might seek someone in a helping profession. You don't have to be on the verge of a crisis to have legitimate reasons for calling someone for counseling. Some of these reasons are:

- Relationship problems
- Job loss
- Death in the family
- Compulsive behaviors
- Problems with substance use

- Being bullied
- Feeling isolated or alienated
- Feeling anxious or depressed
- Problems at work
- Dealing with a chronic illness or pain
- Inability to concentrate
- Forgetfulness
- Lack of meaning or purpose
- Wanting a new career
- Becoming an empty nester
- Infidelity
- A sick or dying parent
- Sexual dysfunction
- Lack of energy
- Inability to relax

This list doesn't even begin to exhaust all of the reasons that someone may want to seek help from a counselor. The point I want to make is that all of us at some point in our lives are going to deal with issues that give us every reason for reaching out. Yes, friends and family can help us, but a trained counselor will have skills that our friends and family members don't. This doesn't mean that we shouldn't talk with our friends and family members about our problems. In fact, it's highly encouraged! We need a strong network of people to get through life. Counselors, however, have specific training that can help people work through problems in a way that's fundamentally different than how we discuss problems with others we're close to.

Who is this book for?

We all can benefit from a better understanding of ourselves. There's no shame in seeking help for anything that you feel is impacting any significant area of your life. It's that simple. Too many of us waste precious time because we don't seek help, or sought help after many years had passed. My wish for this book would be that it sits on a bookshelf in every household so that anyone living there can open it up and discover that there's someone who can lend a hand with life's problems. I want this book to be accessible to those from any background. As a result, I'll attempt to minimize jargon and terms that those without any familiarity with psychology would find foreign.

I also want this book to be accessible to those from any race, religion, sexual orientation, or gender. I'll be writing primarily with those who live in the United States in mind, as that's where I was educated and is the area covered by the various boards and licenses that I'll be writing about.

How to use this book

This book is organized so that you can get a general understanding about the helping professions in several areas. The chapters need not be read in order. If there's any topic you want to learn more about, just skip right to that section. You may find yourself coming back to skipped chapters in the future as needed.

What does it mean to get help?

To seek help from someone in the mental health field, or what we might even call the well-being field, is to take an active step in changing one's life. It's a sign of self-respect and optimism. It's a sign that someone is wise enough to know that with the aid of someone else, they can make their situation better than it currently is.

Some people say disparagingly, "He needs help." Well, he probably does, but so do the people saying it. Implying that getting help should be considered an insult only shows a lack of understanding regarding how much we all can grow from working with those in the helping professions. Those who've benefitted from counseling or therapy have learned that it can be a powerful tool for growth and well-being and not simply a last resort for people whose behaviors are seen by others as problematic.

CHAPTER 3
What is Psychotherapy?

Psychotherapy, or therapy, covers a broad set of theories and activities that typically involve a professional helper working with clients on problems that may relate to emotions, behaviors, thoughts, feelings, and bodily sensations. I'll use the term psychotherapy in this book to be clear that we aren't talking about physical therapy or any other types of therapy. Within the realm of psychotherapy, there's a vast array of methods used that are based upon varying evidence, research, philosophies, and theoretical models. These variations in method and school of thought will be briefly covered later in the book (see Chapter 7). You can think about the differences in psychotherapy approaches as being similar to the differences in musical styles. Jazz and rock 'n' roll might sound drastically different, but we understand both as types of music.

What's important to know is that after decades of study and research, we know that the alliance between the client and the psychotherapist is a more important factor for determining whether therapy is successful than which method is used. As Sperry and Carlson (2013) say, "It is the therapist and not the treatment that influences the amount of therapeutic change that occurs. Relationship skills or developing a therapeutic alliance is the cornerstone of therapeutic excellence."

What this means is that if you're looking for a therapist, what's most significant is how much you feel you can talk with them about what can be deeply personal and intimate topics. In short, a perfect psychotherapy method doesn't exist anymore than a perfect style of music exists. There are likely many psychotherapists from varying schools of thought that you can build a therapeutic alliance with, and the alliance is what's most important when deciding who to work with.

What are the goals of psychotherapy?

I believe the goals of psychotherapy (largely inspired by psychodynamic therapist and professor, Nancy

McWilliams, PhD, ABPP) are to help the client 1) manage stress and their symptoms in healthier ways; 2) understand themselves better, including what their motivations are and how they create relationship patterns in their life; 3) generate meaning in their life; and 4) be able to experience and tolerate a broader range of human emotions.

Our mission as helpers is to support the client while we work on problems, but also to help them develop the skills and self-confidence to, in some ways, become their own therapist as they continue through life. A good therapist wants to help empower the client. A bad therapist wants the client to be dependent on them. That said, a long-term relationship with a counselor can be beneficial as long as both the client and counselor are working in good faith and growth is still occurring. The critical component of determining the quality of the relationship is intent. The intent of a good therapist is to help the client grow out of unhealthy behaviors and maladaptive relational patterns and into a more integrated self. Outside of limitations imposed by insurance companies, the client is ultimately the one who gets to decide whether to stay in therapy, not the helper.

How does psychotherapy work?

The good news is that there's general consensus and evidence that psychotherapy works with most people. However, there is disagreement about exactly how psychotherapy works. Nevertheless, I consider the simplest and clearest understanding of psychotherapy to be one that explains it as being comprised of three general domains: exploration, insight, and action.

When I'm working with a client, we'll always be working on all three areas, but some require more focus than others depending on where we are in our work together. During exploration, I'll get to understand them and their story, needs, and feelings. With insight, I can help shine a light on areas that may have been hidden from them. With action, we'll experiment with ways they can change specific behaviors to help them work toward a life that means something more to them and feels more real and alive than what they're currently experiencing.

Why does psychotherapy work?

There are many theories about exactly why therapy works. A popular one says that there are a few common factors to all types of therapy and those are the main reasons why it works. Some common factors given credit for helping create change are the alliance between client and therapist, empathy, expectations, cultural sensitivity, and collaboration (Wampold 2015). In some ways, we can say that therapy might work when the therapist and client both genuinely care about the process and the two can collaborate on the purpose of the therapy. And yes, the purpose can just be to understand oneself better.

When psychotherapy doesn't work

It's important to know that sometimes psychotherapy doesn't work. Clients have many factors in their lives that impact the therapy. Substance use, missed sessions, motivation, the influence of significant people, and many more factors have a bearing on the outcome. There are no guarantees in therapy. Sometimes the critical areas that must be explored in therapy are too uncomfortable and so clients drop out before the relationship can have a positive effect. While counselors can help their clients cope with the strong feelings that come up in therapy, it's not always the case that people are willing to expose themselves to the emotions that therapy brings up.

CHAPTER 4
The Different Types of Counseling

There are many ways to get help. Deciding what type of help you need is a good place to start if you haven't decided yet.

Individual Counseling

Individual counseling is exactly what you'd think: You sit *individually* with a counselor of some type and work on your life as an individual. Typically, the first session will be an intake where the professional will try to cover at a high level why you're coming in. Each practitioner has their own way of conducting the first session, but it's essentially used to orient each person to the other. After your first session, you can typically expect 45– to 55-minute sessions that explore your presenting issues in more depth. The way problems are addressed will depend on each counselor's approach.

Couples Counseling

You guessed right. Couples counseling involves you and your partner sitting with a professional who will help you work on your relationship. A couple's counselor is trained to help with your relationship dynamics and communication. The intake process will likely be similar to that of individual counseling but with a focus on the relationship, not on each individual's problems (though these inevitably will come up). Session lengths are also likely to be similar to those of individual counseling, 45 to 55 minutes.

Family Therapy

You're getting good at this. Family therapy involves the entire family, or as much of the family that's willing to participate. Common issues that may be addressed include communication problems; family members trying to work out the death of a patriarch or matriarch and the subsequent financial and emotional problems that emerge; the effects of divorce; a recent adoption; or how the severe and persistent mental illness of a family member affects the entire family. Many events and circumstances can lead a family to seek family therapy. Like the other therapy types, family therapy will have an intake process and then follow-up sessions. Because of the larger number of participants, sessions may be longer than individual or couple's sessions. It's reasonable to expect a family therapy session to be 60 to 90 minutes in length.

Group Counseling

You nailed it. Group counseling sessions center on a particular problem that everyone in the group shares. The problems can deal with many topics: PTSD, eating disorders, domestic violence, video game addiction, or any other issue where people seek help and support as a group. Group counseling sessions are different from support groups in that they're led by a professional. Support groups may be formed by people in the general public who may have specific training to lead the support group but may or may not be professionally trained as a counselor.

Addictions Counseling

Addictions can include alcohol and drug use but also gambling, shopping, and other compulsive behaviors. Many times, addictions counseling is a combination of individual therapy and group counseling.

Life Coaching or Coaching

This type of help is typically for those who are otherwise doing well but are looking for someone to help them excel or improve in one or more areas of their life. Life coaches may or may not be licensed counselors or psychologists. Life coaching isn't governed by a professional board, although some professional organizations are emerging. Some of these groups offer training but aren't part of a state licensing board. Health insurance doesn't cover life coaching, and it must be paid for out of pocket.

Career Counseling

Career counseling can be helpful when someone is uncertain about how to take the next step in their career.

Whether the client is a high schooler trying to figure out what to pursue in college or someone with twenty years of experience in their field, a career counselor's job is to help their clients find more meaning in their work.

It's not uncommon to be involved in more than one type of counseling. Someone might be in individual therapy but also in a counseling group. Using the music analogy, this might be like taking private guitar lessons while also rehearsing with a band.

CHAPTER 5
The Different Types of Helpers

Fortunately, the mental health field doesn't have the number of obscure specializations as the medical field does. There are only a few primary types of helpers with varying degrees of education and a different emphasis on what kinds of problems they help with. This chapter explores these roles.

Psychiatrists

Psychiatrists are medical doctors. Psychiatrists will make a diagnosis after meeting with patients and most likely prescribe medication. Although they're able to, psychiatrists typically aren't in the business of conducting lengthy, ongoing psychotherapy with patients. Rather, they'll check in with patients and alter their prescriptions as they see fit, depending on how their patient is doing. As a result, people whose treatment includes both medication and therapy may see both a psychiatrist and a psychotherapist. Psychiatrists' training is mainly grounded in biology, including genetics and neuroscience. As medical doctors, they can order laboratory tests as well as various psychological assessments. Dr. Frasier Crane on the popular TV shows *Cheers* and *Frasier* was a psychiatrist.

Psychologists

Psychologists aren't medical doctors, but they have advanced degrees. Most states require psychologists to have a PhD, PsyD, or similar doctoral-level education. This level of education will typically include a lengthy residency at a mental health facility or in private practice. Psychologists can order and interpret psychological assessments. Many psychologists also conduct regular psychotherapy sessions with patients. Professor Xavier in the *X-Men* franchise was both a psychologist and a psychiatrist.

Counselors

Licensed counselors typically have a master's-level

education. They cannot prescribe medication. They can give many but not all assessments. Licensed counselors typically are highly trained clinical therapists; conducting therapy is their primary responsibility. To become licensed, counselors will also have worked under a supervisor for thousands of hours early in their training. Many people with the title "psychotherapist" are licensed counselors. Depending on the state, LPC or LPCC after someone's name means they are a licensed counselor. Deanna Troi was the counselor on the *USS Enterprise-D* on *Star Trek: The Next Generation*.

Career Counselors

Most career counselors have the same education level and credentials as other counselors. The difference is that career counselors focus on helping people develop their careers rather than on the broader realm of problems. Career counselors will use assessments and models oriented toward their clients' career decisions. In addition, career counselors are keenly aware that there are many factors that can be barriers to someone choosing a career, such as personal relationships and culture. A trained career counselor will not only need to help someone find out what they want to do but also help them deal with all of the other life factors so that they can succeed. Many career counselors are licensed counselors or psychologists.

Addictions Counselors

In the past, addictions counselors didn't need higher education to work in treatment clinics; this type of counselor typically was formerly addicted to a substance and skilled in working with those in recovery. Now, many counselors who deal with drug and alcohol use have a license known as an LADC, or licensed alcohol and drug counselor. LADC typically requires a bachelor's-level education—some may have more education, though. It's not unusual for an addictions counselor to be a licensed professional counselor as well. This dual training means the professional has been trained to do general counseling as well as deal specifically with issues relating to substance use.

Social Workers

Social work requires a master's-level education dealing with issues involving mental and emotional health. Social workers deal frequently with those of low socio-economic status and typically are part of a broader network of helping organizations. If you see LCSW after someone's name, this means they're a licensed social worker. Many times, social workers are involved in the public school system, trying to help children who are living in family situations that may be particularly troubled. They also might be employed in homeless shelters and related organizations. Paige Matthews, played by Rose McGowan on the TV show *Charmed,* became a social worker.

Family Therapist

A licensed family therapist holds a master's-level degree. They've been trained in the particular theories, models, and skills to conduct family therapy. Family therapists will typically have LMFT after their name, depending on what state they're practicing in. *Family Therapy with Dr. Jenn* on VH-1 depicts a family therapist.

Psychotherapists

"Psychotherapist" can be thought of as a generic term and isn't protected by a licensing board in most states. The term implies that someone is trained in counseling, psychology, and the field's theories and models. It's not unusual for licensed counselors to refer to themselves as psychotherapists.

Life Coaches or Coaches

The title "coach" doesn't imply any particular training or licensing. Life coaching isn't governed by a professional state licensing board like those that govern psychiatrists, psychologists, licensed counselors, social workers, and marriage and family therapists. Anyone can call themselves a life coach. This doesn't mean the person can't be helpful—just be wary since no professional training or testing is required to be a coach.

CHAPTER 6
Types of Mental Health Organizations

Mental health organizations come in many shapes and sizes. Some provide a wide range of services, while others specialize in only one type of treatment, like substance use or children's mental health. The quality of an organization can't be determined by its size or how many services it offers. The culture, policies, and practitioners will largely determine how much value the business provides.

Private Practice

A private practice is a common type of organization that provides mental health services. Typically, one or two therapists (sometimes more) share a space in an office center or a converted home. Very often, private practices are one-person operations. Therapists open private practices for many reasons, but most of the time it's to have more flexibility and control over their schedule. Being in private practice isn't easy, so many don't do it.

The pros of going to a private practice are that the chances of working with the same therapist throughout your treatment is high. If you have a good relationship with the counselor, you'll work together as long as you're in treatment, unless they retire or quit practicing. In other organizations, you may see different counselors throughout your treatment. This isn't necessarily a problem, but since the therapeutic alliance is one of the most important factors that determine successful therapy, seeing the same therapist is a definite plus. A private practice also may be more flexible with payment terms, such as offering a more generous sliding scale or deferring payment for a period of time if you encounter financial problems.

There are some cons to going to a private practice. Since a private practice can be just one person, the hours of operation are tied to the schedule of that person. If the therapist goes on vacation for a while, you will likely have to go to a different practice if you're in crisis and need to talk with someone while your primary therapist is away. This backup person might be provided to you by your primary therapist but not necessarily. Another con of going to a private practice is that it may not accept as many insurance plans as larger clinics or have limited payment options.

Mental Health Clinic

Mental health clinics are larger organizations with many therapists, professionals, and support staff. These can vary in size, with perhaps five to ten counselors, while even larger ones may be affiliated with a hospital network or other large medical affiliation.

The pros and cons of a mental health clinic are essentially the opposite of a private practice. A mental health clinic will have many counselors working, so you can generally make an appointment for a time that's more convenient than if you were going to a private practice. By going to a mental health clinic, you're more likely to be seen sooner. Mental health clinics may accept a wider range of insurance than certain private practices.

However, mental health clinics have much higher employee turnover than private practices. It's much more likely that your therapist at a mental health clinic will move on to a different job or open their own private practice during the course of treatment. Mental health clinics will typically not offer as flexible a sliding scale if you don't have insurance. They're also probably not going to be as flexible if you miss a payment or are having prolonged financial hardship.

In-patient

In-patient clinics treat people who need to stay at the facility for a period of time because of the severity of their condition. Most of the time, people seek in-patient treatment for substance use problems. However, people may also need to seek in-patient treatment for other problems such as being a threat to themselves or having a psychotic episode.

For obvious reasons, in-patient treatment is one of the most expensive types of treatments for mental health. Because housing, living, security, and staffing costs are incurred, in-patient facilities must charge much higher rates for services. Insurance companies have their own policies for what in-patient treatment they'll pay for. If you're considering in-patient treatment for yourself or a loved one, check with your insurance company to determine what they'll pay for and what clinics are in their network for your policy. Unfortunately, without insurance, in-patient treatment is prohibitively expensive for most people.

Out-patient

Out-patient treatment simply means that the person seeking treatment leaves the facility each day when treatment is over. Out-patient treatment can include programs that are more intensive than meeting with a counselor each week. The sessions may be longer, even half a day or longer, and may meet more than once per week. They may also include individual and group counseling. Substance use problems are one of the most common reasons why people seek this type of mental health treatment organization.

CHAPTER 7
Treatment Approaches

There are more treatment approaches than I can fit within the scope of this book. While I'll try to paint a broad picture of the many categories and the theories and research behind them, each particular treatment approach likely has various branches and subgroups that won't be covered in this chapter—it would be as difficult and lengthy as detailing the differences in musical subgenres.

Experiential

Experiential psychotherapy focuses on the experiences that happen during the session. This means focusing on feelings and emotions and being guided past psychological defenses that keep you from experiencing certain emotions. Emotions provide important information and a vitality to life; experiential therapy helps bring these to consciousness.

Psychoanalytic and Psychodynamic

Psychoanalytic and psychodynamic models have their roots in the theories of Sigmund Freud, the father of psychoanalysis. Many of Freud's ideas aren't used in treatment, though, and almost all of modern psychoanalytic treatment wouldn't be recognizable to the originator. There's a long history of this type of treatment that influences how practically all therapists conceptualize how humans think and feel.

This treatment focuses on the therapist trying to help you understand yourself better. The therapist will want to explore the relationships you have with your family and significant others as well as significant events in your past. The therapist will look at how the two of you interact and try to provide insight into how old patterns may be interfering in your present life. This approach explores what has meaning for you and helps to expand the range of emotional experience. This style of treatment is very deep and broad philosophically. There are many different approaches used by those who fall under this umbrella of treatment, but they all have in common the use of certain psychoanalytic concepts and techniques.

Behavioral and Cognitive

Those who practice this type of therapy typically focus on looking at thought patterns and how to change them. Goals are typically related to changing specific behaviors. Do you get angry every time you drive? A cognitive behaviorist will try to examine the process—when you start getting angry, how it gets triggered or escalates—and how to change that process. This approach also focuses on examining untrue beliefs about oneself and the world and how they affect feelings and behaviors. Timelines are short-term compared to many other techniques.

Existential and Humanistic

Existential and humanistic approaches deal with fundamental aspects of being human. Many times, this involves finding meaning and purpose in our lives. These approaches also deal with our mortality and making the most of our time on earth. Through this approach, we seek to have more enriched lives, living with purpose, and seeking meaningful connection with those around us.

Neuroscientific

This approach centers on how the scientific community currently understands the functioning of the brain. The neuropsychotherapist still helps the client deal with presenting problems using fundamental counseling approaches, but they also help the client understand how the brain works and ways to leverage that to try to remedy problems. A neuroscientific approach can be thought of as an add-on to other treatments since it still depends on using counseling techniques from other models.

Integrated

There are very few purists in the field of psychotherapy. What I mean by that is that most therapists are influenced by many models and theories. This is what is known as an integrated, or eclectic, approach. If a therapist lists many treatment approaches, they're using an eclectic treatment approach. If a therapist says they use an integrated or eclectic approach, they should still be able to articulate the different models they use and why. Someone who can't tell you the details of the models they've integrated and how they use them might not be clear in what they're doing. Be wary of someone using an integrated or eclectic approach who doesn't have a clear answer to the question, "Please tell me what models you've integrated and how you use them."

CHAPTER 8
Types of Problems

There are many symptoms, experiences, and behaviors that lead people to therapy. Life, even when it's at its best, can be tough. Talking with a mental health counselor during challenging times is perfectly reasonable. While the problems listed in this chapter aren't exhaustive, they illustrate how much we all have to deal with and how normal it is to seek help. In fact, notice that I purposely don't go into detail regarding severe and persistent mental illnesses that many times require the intervention of a psychiatrist. The reason for this decision is to hopefully illuminate the fact that even people who are functioning in everyday society struggle. This type of mundane struggle with life can be helped with counseling and psychotherapy when there's a clinically significant impact.

Addictions

To expand on common struggles, many people, if not

most, are addicted to something. Whether legal or illegal drugs, sex, gambling, food, smartphones, or something else, anything you do more often than you'd like is suitable to bring up with a counselor. It's a misperception that someone has to be strung-out in an alley before they should see someone for help. If you have a behavior that you want to change, a therapist can help.

Anxiety and Depression

Anxiety and depression are very common symptoms that counselors help with. There's a wide range of severity of most symptoms. Whether you feel on edge or are having full-blown panic attacks, this anxiety can be treated with therapy. Similarly, whether one feels down more often that they'd like or whether they struggle to even get out of bed, depression is commonly treated with psychotherapy.

Autism and Child Development

Autism, which now includes what was once called Asperger's syndrome, can be helped with therapy, particularly certain types of neurofeedback therapy. However, those with autism may also struggle with relationships, and a therapist can help them relate better to others.

Child development and parenting concerns are many times first explored with a pediatrician. However, pediatricians may refer parents to a counselor to work through stress, anxiety, depression, and other problems that occur during childhood. If a child seems to be overwhelmed by particular feelings, a child psychologist or psychotherapist can help.

Eating Disorders

Struggling to maintain a healthy weight or suffering from eating disorders can be eased with therapy. Many times, a deficit of emotional regulation or the side effects of trauma relate to problems in this area. Many therapists specialize in dealing with eating disorders of all types.

Trauma

Trauma comes in many forms, such as being

involved in a car crash or a child witnessing domestic violence. Sometimes symptoms of trauma aren't easily noticed by the individual. Signs of trauma include feeling numb, being very alert, feelings of helplessness, and more. Therapists frequently encounter clients who've experienced trauma.

Grief

At some point in everyone's life, they will experience loss. Dealing with grief can be terrible, even with a strong support group. Counselors can help you deal with grief and loss to help you get through any of life's inevitable tragedies.

Existential Issues

Happiness and having purpose and meaning are important in life. Counselors can help someone discover what they want to get out of life, including exploring identity. This usually involves examining one's values and finding out if the client is living accordingly. It can also include an exploration of spirituality, which for many is intertwined with happiness and meaning. A therapist who says they deal with existential issues is referring to all of these topics.

Sleep and Stress

Quality sleep, health, work-life balance, and stress are intertwined. If you aren't getting enough sleep, life can be more stressful and affect health. Having enough time throughout the week to decompress from work and responsibility is important. Therapists can examine problem areas and help find solutions so that physical and mental health are working in sync.

Personality

Personality problems can make life very challenging. Those who avoid others, treat others poorly, or have any of the many personality problems that can be treated with psychotherapy will hopefully find life much more enjoyable once they have insight into how they interact with others and why others may react the way they do.

Personality problems can take some time to address in therapy since so much of our personalities are wrapped up in our identities. Even though this type of therapy can move slowly at times, without knowing how others see us and how we create our own problems, we will always struggle unnecessarily in some areas.

Relationships

Relationships are essential to healthy emotions. We are social creatures, and we need good relationships to live life fully. Working with a counselor is a relational experience. Much about how we relate to others can be learned by entering counseling. While some issues are more difficult to treat with counseling, helping with relational problems is an area where psychotherapy shines.

CHAPTER 9
How to Find a Therapist

Some people give up on getting help because they aren't sure how to find someone. If you have health insurance, most plans have mental health benefits. Calling your insurance company to find out what therapists are in its network is a great place to start. If you find a therapist some other way, you'll likely need to check with your insurance company anyway, so why not start with them before beginning your search? If you're paying out of pocket, then you'll obviously skip the step that involves contacting an insurance company.

Internet Profiles

Unless you have a referral from a friend, family member, or doctor, you're probably hunting on your own to find someone who can help. Most people today find their therapist using a search engine or other internet resource. If you're using a search engine, many of the highest results will lead you to psychotherapy websites where thousands of therapists have profiles. Not only can the number of results be overwhelming if you're in the city, or underwhelming if you aren't, they can be completely confusing no matter where you live. I often wonder who these listing websites think their audience is: psychotherapists, or the people seeking help? If I didn't have an advanced degree in counseling, I honestly wouldn't know what most of the content on therapist profiles meant or why I should care.

Psychodynamic, neuropsychotherapist, cognitive behavioral, emotionally focused—for most people looking to find a therapist, these words only serve to make it more frustrating or scary rather than warm and welcoming. This is where I want to gently remind you that the therapists themselves are more important than the type of therapy. In other words, finding a therapist that you feel good about working with is more important that finding a therapist that has the one perfect treatment orientation. And don't expect to find the one perfect therapist for your problems—because they don't exist.

A Good Therapist Match

Some therapists claim competency in almost every sort of mental health issue that exists. It's not uncommon to come across an internet listing of a therapist that requires a bit of scrolling to see all of the symptoms that they treat. While many therapists have treated almost every symptom out there in the course of their professional work, it doesn't hurt to look for people who specialize in a particular area in some cases.

For example, seeing a therapist who specializes in trauma can be a good idea if you've suffered a traumatic childhood or event. Someone with schizophrenia will likely want to work with someone who specializes in that area. This is where looking for a therapist isn't entirely unlike finding someone to work on your car. If you just need an oil change or maintenance, then there are plenty of therapists who do a great job. However, for an exotic model, you'll probably want to find a specialty shop.

Psychotherapy isn't magic. It's applying methods in the context of a trusting relationship between a patient and a therapist. Building trust is the critical factor, and that's why not every patient will succeed with just any therapist. We all have different triggers, and we need to work with someone we feel we can open up to.

The important thing to remember about finding a good psychotherapy match is that if a patient and therapist can forge trust, then progress can be made using practically any of the techniques available. Therapists tend to employ only the techniques they find value in, and many times those are the techniques that match their personality. Therefore, if you and your therapist are a good personality match, then the techniques they use stand a good chance of being well-received by you as well.

CHAPTER 10
Insurance and Payment Terms

Payment Terms

Payment terms will vary from practice to practice. Methods of payment may include cash, credit card, check, or insurance. The ethical guidelines around bartering aren't black and white. While bartering can be an option, it introduces what can be a tricky situation around boundaries and potential exploitation—consider this option carefully.

Private Pay

There are reasons you may prefer to pay out of pocket for your sessions if you can afford it. Insurance companies may limit the number of sessions you may receive, even if you feel like you still require more treatment. Other reasons you may want to pay out of pocket include wanting more privacy, taking the work more seriously, and feeling like you're more invested in the treatment.

Insurance

Practitioners can only accept insurance from companies where they're credentialed. Not only is this process complicated for therapists, but it complicates their ability to provide services to the general public. Each state typically has many different third-party payers, or insurance companies. Most counselors only accept some of them. Keep in mind, many therapists would accept more types of insurance, but it's up to the insurance company to allow particular therapists to be in their network. Since insurance companies decide which counselors they'll reimburse, there's no guarantee that the counselor you want to see accepts your insurance. Before making an appointment, always check with the clinic or therapist to be sure that your insurance will be accepted.

Your therapist may know some details of your coverage, but it's not possible for counselors to know the details of every plan provided by every insurer unless they have a sophisticated billing system in the practice.

Many smaller practices have outside companies to do their billing and will not have this information available until after submitting the first claim. If you don't know the details of out-of-pocket costs and co-pays, many times your therapist or their billing person can find this out for you by calling your insurance company.

In-Network

If your insurance provider says that your therapist or counselor is in-network, then depending on the specifics of your policy, sessions will be covered by your insurance company to some extent. Most in-network plans require that your deductible be met before paying any benefits. Once your plan's deductible is met, then your insurance company will begin covering some percentage of your session costs. This can be the entire amount or a percentage—again, it depends on your specific plan.

It's also possible that an in-network plan will require a co-pay for each visit. This usually runs between $20 and $50 and will be paid directly to the therapist at the time of the session.

Out-of-Network

Therapists who aren't credentialed with an insurance company may still be able to bill as an out-of-network provider. If a therapist bills your insurance company as an out-of-network provider, you'll likely have to meet a higher deductible before the insurance company pays any benefits. Sometimes this can be quite high, so always know whether your provider is out-of-network for your plan and how much your out-of-network deductible is.

While a high out-of-network deductible may make it seem like a waste of time to have your therapist bill your insurance company, it can make a difference. If, in an unfortunate year, you have a medical emergency that requires treatment out of network, the out-of-network benefits you've billed for your therapy sessions will have counted toward your out-of-network deductible. If a medical emergency's cost exceeds your out-of-network deductible, you'll want every penny that you paid to count toward it.

Sliding Scale

Most therapists offer what is known as a sliding scale. A therapist's regular rate may be $150 or more per session. However, they may offer a sliding scale that allows those with financial difficulty or without insurance to pay less (in some cases, much less).

Therapists aren't obligated to offer a sliding scale. They do it because they believe in giving help to those who are struggling financially. If a therapist doesn't offer a sliding scale, it doesn't mean they're an uncaring person; they may have many justifiable reasons for not doing so. They may be struggling financially at the moment and might not be able to afford offering a discount on their sessions. Also, because of contracts with insurance companies, providers many times are limited in what sliding scale payments they can offer.

Some therapists use the honor system when offering a sliding scale to clients. They may simply ask the client what they can afford and accept that. However, some therapists may ask for pay stubs or other proof of hardship before consenting to a lower fee. Again, this policy is up to the therapist or clinic to decide.

Pro Bono

Some therapists and clinics may offer free sessions to some clients. Some therapists set aside a certain number of hours each week to see clients for free or for a very low fee. The decision to do this is usually very personal for the therapist. They likely believe strongly that those suffering financial hardships are many times the ones who need counseling the most. These therapists typically have a deep commitment to easing suffering and want to make some of their time available to those with little to no means.

Sometimes therapists will still ask for a token payment of several dollars from those clients who are going through difficult times. The reason is a therapeutic one: Counselors know that clients need to be committed to therapy for it work and that the client must work harder than the therapist to have meaningful results. By asking a person with little to no financial means to still pay a few dollars, they're trying to increase the client's commitment to the therapeutic process.

The important thing to remember about payment is that therapists need to be able to make a living so that they can offer services to the public. They have families to take care of and bills to pay. Therapists typically are paid modestly from performing therapy and have invested many hours in education and ongoing training. Most therapists genuinely care about their clients. The saying goes, "You pay me for my time, but you don't pay me to care. That part is free."

CHAPTER 11
Multicultural Issues

For most of counseling's history in America, issues relating to differences between cultures were largely ignored. It wasn't until 1995 that the American Counseling Association's code of ethics substantially addressed multiculturalism. As a result, there are many counselors still practicing who were trained prior the emphasis on having an ethical duty to be culturally sensitive. This isn't meant to imply that those counselors aren't sensitive to diverse cultures, only to state the facts regarding how recently multiculturalism has been formally adopted as part of counselor training. Now counselors receive this type of training in the standard curriculum.

Counselors are trained not to impose their values or worldview on clients. The goal of therapy isn't to turn a client into a version of the psychotherapist; the point is to help foster psychological health and behavioral health in their many forms, not to prescribe ideologies and cultural beliefs. Prospective clients who aren't from the dominant culture must be able to receive therapy from a counselor with a different background and have their culture, sexual orientation, and religious beliefs respected and left intact, so long as that's what the client decides. (It's not unusual for long-held beliefs to change during the course of therapy, which may include alterations to religious beliefs, sexual identity, and more.)

One of the difficulties for clients who are in a nondominant culture is not being able to easily find therapists who understand their background. In Minnesota, where I live and practice, the statistically average therapist is a white woman in her early 40s who practices in the urban Twin Cities. Obviously, this statistical average is unlike the vast majority of people not only in the Twin Cities but in the entire state. Because the demographic range of therapists is so narrow, if counselors weren't trained in multiculturalism, they wouldn't be able to help most people who come to them. Since the therapeutic alliance is so critical to producing positive outcomes, counselors need to listen carefully to each person who comes to them so that they may respect diversity in all its forms.

The flip side of being sensitive to diversity is being too focused on cultural differences at the expense of seeing the individual. Each person is unique and must be listened to individually. If counselors only see the cultural, religious, racial, and sexual orientation differences, then stereotyping may result. It's imperative that counselors treat the person, not the demographics.

CHAPTER 12
Licenses, Boards, and Ethics

Licenses

A mental health professional with a license typically has had more training, is being held to higher ethical standards, and has much more to lose for behaving badly than someone without a license. This doesn't mean that those without licenses can't help. It just means that you should be aware that if you work with someone who is unlicensed, they won't have been through as rigorous of a process as someone who is. They also won't have to undergo ongoing training or be held accountable for improper professional behavior—and that means something.

In the process of gaining a license, mental health professionals may still be practicing, but under the supervision of someone who is licensed. In these cases, the counselor will inform you at the beginning of treatment that they aren't licensed but are under supervision while pursing one. This situation is common and shouldn't raise any red flags.

Boards

The primary job of a licensing board is to protect the public. Licensing boards exist for each type of license. The boards create codes of ethics and determine whether professionals have violated those ethics when cases are brought to them. State legislatures determine what licenses are valid in that state and what the requirements are for being licensed. In Minnesota, the legislature has passed laws that determine what licenses I can pursue with my master's-level degree. If I move to another state, I may have to apply for a different type of license depending on what that state's legislative body has decided.

Ethics

Ethics are codes of conduct created by boards to hold licensed professionals to a standard of conduct. These codes of conduct are to protect you, the client, first and foremost. The codes are also designed to protect the profession and its standing with the public. If people don't feel like they're safe in a counseling situation, they won't seek counseling. This is why seeing licensed professionals (or those under the supervision of a licensed professional) is almost always a better idea than seeing unlicensed ones.

Ethics in counseling deal with many issues, but in general, they're based on simple but powerful sets of fundamental values and principles. Values can be thought of as ideas that guide interactions between people. Principles can be thought of as more objective ideas that guide the spirit of counseling regardless of who's involved. Not all helpers work according to the same code of ethics (psychologists, social workers, and counselors use different codes), but the spirit of those codes is essentially the same.

The values for those professionals working according to the American Counseling Association's code of ethics (American Counseling Association, 2014) are:

1. Enhancing human development throughout the life span;

2. Honoring diversity and embracing a multicultural approach in support of the worth, dignity, potential, and uniqueness of people within their social and cultural contexts;

3. Promoting social justice;

4. Safeguarding the integrity of the counselor–client relationship; and

5. Practicing in a competent and ethical manner.

These are the principles for those working according to the American Counseling Association's code of ethics (American Counseling Association, 2014):

• *Autonomy*, or fostering the right to control the direction of one's life;

• *Nonmaleficence*, or avoiding actions that cause harm;

• *Beneficence*, or working for the good of the individual and society by promoting mental health and well-being;

• *Justice*, or treating individuals equitably and fostering fairness and equality;

• *Fidelity*, or honoring commitments and keeping promises, including fulfilling one's responsibilities of trust in professional relationships; and

• *Veracity*, or dealing truthfully with individuals with whom counselors come into professional contact.

The actual code of ethics for the ACA covers many specific behaviors and issues, but some of the most important ones relate to client confidentiality and the relationship of the counselor to the client. Therapists are forbidden from sharing the content of your sessions with others. Some exceptions to this are discussing your case with a supervisor or intervening if you are an imminent threat to yourself or someone else. Therapists are also forbidden from exploiting the relationship that you have for personal gain. Examples of this would be asking a client to run errands or doing business together outside of therapy.

I can't emphasize enough how the ethical code that a helper works under protects the client in almost every way. Counselors have a duty to put your well-being first. If you feel that you've been taken advantage of or abused by a helper, contact the board for whatever license the helper has. This is another reminder of why it's important to only work with licensed helpers or those working under the supervision of a licensed therapist. If you feel that you've been treated unethically by an unlicensed helper, there's no board to turn to.

CHAPTER 13
Screenings and Assessments

You might feel overwhelmed or nervous if your therapist asks you if you're ok with taking an assessment or using a screening tool. Hopefully, the information in this chapter will help explain why they're used and how they can be helpful. Both screening tools and assessments can provide the counselor with valuable information that can be used to improve therapy.

Screenings

It's common for a therapist to use a screening early on in your work together. After initially listening to your concerns and learning why you're meeting with the counselor, they may ask you to fill out a questionnaire. These screening tools help the therapist understand how serious a problem is. The forms therapists use have been researched and found to be reliable.

Many different screening tools exist because they're designed to screen for specific problems. For example, the Beck Depression Inventory screens for depression. The Columbia-Suicide Severity Rating Scale assesses risk of suicide. There are screening tools for substance use, pornography use, post-traumatic stress disorder, anxiety, and many, many more.

Screenings are usually brief. They aren't intended to wear you out but rather designed to ask only as many questions needed for the counselor to understand the problem better. Typically, the screening will be done in the counselor's office during a session. They can be quickly scored, but typically the therapist will do this after your session and then discuss the results in the next session.

A detailed example of a screening tool is the CAGE questionnaire. It's a very simple tool used to assess someone for the possibility of excessive drinking. The screening tool only has four questions, all of which have yes-or-no answers. The therapist can pose them directly to the client. Based on how the client responds, the therapist knows whether to explore the issue in more detail.

The CAGE questionnaire is very brief, but even longer screening tools usually aren't more than 10 to 20 questions. The Life Event Checklist screens for the potential existence of trauma and is only 17 items. The Mood Disorder Questionnaire has 13 questions and is used to check for the existence of symptoms that relate to bipolar disorder.

Even though these screenings can have scary names, therapists aren't asking you take them to scare you. Counselors are trained to see you as a whole person and not just as a collection of symptoms or problems. They're asking you to take a screening questionnaire because the information can be valuable in helping you. A counselor or therapist should never treat you with any less respect or dignity based upon the results of a screening tool. They don't want you to take the screening tool to humiliate you; they want you to take it so they can better help you.

Assessments

Assessments are used to try to provide your clinician

with a better view into your personality and who you are. Compared to screening tools, assessments are typically longer and more involved. They're intended to be more comprehensive than screenings, which typically look for the presence of one particular type of symptom. While it can be intimidating to think about taking an assessment and having someone know more about the results than you do, a good clinician will work through the results with you and explain what they mean. There are many types of assessments designed to measure different aspects of the human mind. Depending on the type of help you seek, assessments may not be used at all.

The most common psychological exam that's used to try and find mental health issues is the Minnesota Multiphasic Personality Inventory, or MMPI. It's a bit of a long exam and may take an hour or two to finish. It's been researched heavily and is a reliable instrument for finding problems such as high anxiety, depression, and other issues. Another exam that's used for similar purposes is the Millon Clinical Multiaxial Inventory.

If you take either of these exams, your clinician or a

psychologist who specializes in scoring these assessments will interpret the results. The goal of this process isn't to shame you or to pick you apart but to understand the areas that can be focused on to help you have a better life.

You might wonder how all of this works. Without getting too much into the details and the statistics used to create assessments, one way of looking at your results is to see how they compare to everyone else who has taken the assessment. Assessments don't have right and wrong answers. Assessments are designed to measure specific things, called factors. Some questions might be designed to find the presence of anxiety. Well, everyone has some anxiety—it's just a matter of how much you have compared to everyone else. If your answers indicate a presence of anxiety that's much greater than the average, then the clinician knows that your anxiety is probably much higher than the average person's and is likely causing you more trouble than the average person.

Psychological tests don't always try to find things that are troubling someone. Many of them are designed to find strengths and positive characteristics. Some assessments measure intelligence. Some measure what type of personality you have. If you see a career counselor, you'll almost certainly be asked to take one or more assessments that try to discover what your strengths are, what you're interested in, and how you like to work. These assessments are all designed to help find out what type of work you may be best suited for. Some assessments, like the Strong Interest Inventory, even tell you how your answers match with the professions of others who have taken the test. For example, when I took the assessment, my answers resembled those who are musicians more than any other profession. In fact, I couldn't have scored any more similar to the musicians who took it. (And yes, I am a musician as well as a counselor.)

CHAPTER 14
Telepsychotherapy

In the simplest terms, telepsychotherapy can be defined as any communications that occur remotely using technology for the purpose of conducting psychotherapy. *Tele* is Greek for "from a distance." Subsequently, telepsychotherapy can also be thought of as any psychotherapy conducted from a distance. Electronic communications of all types may aid in telepsychotherapy. This includes the use of HIPPA-compliant video conferencing, email, and more. Independent of any particular theoretical orientation, any communications using these and other internet-based technologies for the purpose of performing psychotherapy can be considered telepsychotherapy.

The reason telepsychotherapy has been adopted so quickly is that it has some strengths compared to face-to-face counseling. If telepsychotherapy didn't have characteristics that made it preferable to in-person counseling in some scenarios, then it certainly wouldn't be used to the extent it is. Finn and Barak (2010) say that studies have found that online therapy results in successful therapeutic alliances at the same rate as in-person counseling. They also say that studies report that consumer satisfaction with online therapy is similar to face-to-face consumer satisfaction. As a result, there's no reason to believe that telepsychotherapy suffers from a deficit of the most basic element necessary for counseling to work.

Even in the beginning years of widespread internet adoption, counseling professionals saw the merits of using technology in certain areas. Oravec (2000) wrote that the use of technology with families can eliminate one of the most significant barriers that prevents them from entering counseling: scheduling. Once the number of people who are required to meet at the same place and same time grows, the difficulty in scheduling can become so enormous that some families simply give up on going. One of the strengths of telepsychotherapy is that it enables families to use remote technology to more conveniently meet online with a family therapist.

Li, Jaladin, and Abdullah (2013) discuss the usefulness of using telepsychotherapy as a way to intervene when clients suffer from social phobia. They explain that even those who have no social phobia but who have a fear of the social stigma of attending therapy could potentially benefit from telepsychotherapy since no one would see them entering a therapist's office. Having a means of providing privacy in this way can be even more important in small towns or rural areas where people tend to know each other more.

Rummell and Joyce (2010) say that one strength of telepsychotherapy is that it makes practitioners who specialize in a specific area of treatment available to those in more geographic areas. For example, a client may suffer from a seldom-treated diagnosis. With the use of telepsychotherapy, the client may be able to benefit from the expertise of a therapist who specializes in that disorder but who practices in a faraway location.

Counselors using telepsychotherapy must follow the same ethical principles as when operating face-to-face. Nevertheless, technology presents counselors with unique scenarios that require new ways of thinking about how to ethically conduct treatment. The anonymity of the internet can be both a strength and a weakness of using it for therapy. While it can be a gift to those suffering from anxieties and issues that are made worse by being in public, such as those who suffer from agoraphobia and social anxiety, verifying a person's identity can be an issue if circumstances require intervening at the client's physical location. While anonymity isn't the only characteristic of telepsychotherapy that raises ethical issues, it seems to raise many of the most serious ones.

Therapists' attitudes toward telepsychotherapy vary across demographics. Research surveys suggest that telepsychotherapy is generally seen as useful, at least in some capacity. Most therapists must use at least some technology in their practice. As a result, therapists seem to want to learn more about technology and how to use it at work. Nevertheless, telepsychotherapy doesn't seem to be a serious alternative to meeting with clients in-person. As a result, counselors will still primarily be using in-person therapy for the foreseeable future.

Rules around licensing when doing telepsychotherapy are tricky. Since state legislatures typically create the laws around telepsychotherapy, they vary across the country. It's the responsibility of your therapist to know whether they're violating any laws or regulations when working across state lines.

CHAPTER 15
Problems That Can Arise

Therapists are human and come with their own problems. Like any relationship, sometimes things can go wrong between therapist and client. This isn't necessarily a bad thing. Learning to deal with a relationship rupture is a critical skill that everyone needs. After a rupture, a relationship can be repaired and become stronger. Moving through this process with a counselor can help people learn to repair relationships in their personal lives. Nevertheless, you need to understand some of the common issues that can arise.

Problems that can typically be resolved

Most problems that come up in counseling can be resolved if each person wants the relationship to continue. Common problems in therapy include:

Finding convenient scheduling options. Not all therapists schedule clients the same way. Some have dedicated times for each client; others have a calendar that gets filled on a first-come, first-served basis. You'll have to learn how each therapist does their scheduling and schedule sessions in a way that works for both parties.

Insurance snafus. If your therapist accepts insurance, there might be times that things crop up that need to be dealt with. Don't be concerned if at the beginning of a session your therapist needs to handle an administrative insurance task with you.

Therapist vacations. Counseling is a tough job, and therapists need time to recharge. A good therapist will let you know well in advance of upcoming vacations so you can prepare. They might also leave you with the contact information of a backup therapist you can contact while they're away.

Disagreements. Not that it should have to happen or happen regularly, but it's normal for you to disagree with your therapist. If you disagree with something your therapist says, let them know. They should want to understand why you feel the way you do and talk through the differences.

Different cultural or spiritual backgrounds between counselor and client. Navigating different cultural backgrounds can present a challenge from time to time. However, counselors are trained to be culturally sensitive, and they're ethically required to respect cultural differences.

Problems that might be tougher to solve

Inability to pay. Therapists do care about your outcome in therapy and want you to get better. That said, counselors can't stay in business if they don't have an income—they also need to pay bills, both personal and business related. That income either has to come from third-party payers, such as insurance companies, or from the client in the form of cash payments. If, for whatever reason, you can no longer afford therapy and you don't have insurance, your therapist might agree to a reduction in fees until your situation improves. Nevertheless, if you're unable to pay at all, at some point in time your counselor will likely need to refer you to a free counseling center or somewhere else that's willing to see you at no cost.

You don't trust your counselor. If you've worked with your counselor for some time and you don't feel you can trust them, then you should find someone else. The therapeutic alliance is critical for therapy to work. If there's no alliance, then you're wasting your time seeing that particular therapist, whether they're actually trustworthy or not. There are many reasons why you might not trust your therapist to help you. You might feel like they don't listen or that they don't have enough competency with your particular problem. That being said, if you're someone who doesn't trust people in general, then learning to trust someone is something critical that must be worked on. If you never give a counselor the chance to help you, then you'll always be let down.

Problems that require seeing another counselor

An abusive counselor. Fortunately, this doesn't happen

often, but it does happen. During my training, I heard over and over again that the one and only clear-cut mistake a counselor can make is to have a sexual relationship with a client. Nevertheless, I was told that at some point in my career, I will hear about one of my colleagues who had to go before the board because they slept with a client. If, for whatever reason, this happens to you in the course of counseling, you need to know that it's always inappropriate and you should stop seeing the therapist immediately.

CHAPTER 16
Ending Counseling

While there's nothing wrong with seeing a counselor each week for many years, or even until the end of one's life, the goal of therapy isn't for the client to be dependent upon the therapist but to understand themselves and be able to deal with life's problems—not alone, but with meaningful connections and the psychological skills that are learned through the course of therapy.

Different orientations tend to vary greatly in their opinions regarding how long therapy should last. Psychoanalytic and psychodynamic orientations have no qualms about someone being in therapy for years. After all, uncovering the many layers of one's childhood and psychological processes can't be done in a few hours. However, it's not unusual for a cognitive behavioral therapist to treat a particular symptom, such as a phobia, in fewer than ten sessions. The important point is: *How long you're in therapy isn't up to the therapist, it's up to you (or your insurance company if you aren't paying out-of-pocket).*

In earlier chapters, we went through the different orientations and discussed a little bit about each approach to therapy. Whichever approach sounds like a good fit for you is the one you might want to do. There's no evidence that any one approach is more effective than any other. I'm repeating this because I want you to feel empowered about not only choosing which type of help you get but when to decide to finish it. Life will always be problematic; the goal of therapy isn't to solve all of your problems. In fact, no one can tell you what the goal of your therapy is because *you* decide what the goal of your therapy is. If you want to have better relationships with your children and through the course of therapy you gain that, then your initial goal has been met. If you decide to work on something else, that's your decision, but it's also your decision to end counseling.

Not only are you the one to decide what the goal of your therapy should be, but you get to decide when and whether it's been attained. That being said, there's nothing wrong with asking your therapist their opinion regarding progress and further opportunities for exploration. They should have insight and ideas about furthering your work together if you feel like it's something you want to continue.

What I'm cautioning against is the feeling that you must be in therapy for lengthy periods of time or that you can only be helped by one particular therapist. There are many, many helpers out there. No one should feel like there's only one counselor in the world that can understand them or that if they leave therapy that their lives will fall apart. If you feel that way after being in a lengthy counseling relationship, that may very well be a warning sign that something isn't working.

When the time comes and you decide that you want to end counseling, bring it up to your therapist. You'll likely want one or more sessions to process the entirety of your work together. I don't recommend quitting therapy abruptly unless you feel you have been in an abusive relationship with your helper. (Then, by all means, leave abruptly.)

There will also be circumstances where you don't get to decide to end therapy. Counselors have many reasons for ending the therapeutic relationship. They may retire because of age, health, or both. They may take a new job or move to another state. Counselors can also end treatment if they feel that they aren't able to help you for whatever reason. This doesn't happen often, but it does happen. If your therapist concludes treatment for any reason, they should provide you with referrals.

The end of therapy can feel overwhelming if you've been in a counseling relationship with someone for a long time. To be helped can leave someone with a deep feeling of gratitude and a deep feeling of loss knowing that a special relationship will soon be over. But with a good dose of hope, you'll move into a new part of your life, having been listened to, respected, treated with dignity, and helped.

CHAPTER 17
Final Words

The purpose of this book isn't to push any one type of therapy but to help you understand the mental health field so that it's less scary and so that using it is less stigmatizing. If I could have everyone who reads this book take away one thing, it would be to believe that your life might get better by working with a therapist you like.

Without treating yourself well—with love, dignity, and respect—you can't extend the same generosity to others. Many helping relationships aim to support you in doing just that. Learning to treat yourself differently than you do now, after years of life's wear and tear, takes time. Please be patient with yourself and the process.

I want to encourage you to not give up on yourself. Everyone encounters difficulties during life, and it's never any better going through them alone. Please give someone a chance to help you.

Take care,

APPENDIX
Questions to Ask a Potential Therapist

The questions that follow are intended to help you get a feel for how your therapist might work with you. What you want to consider is whether the way your therapist works sounds appealing to you. There are many ways to do therapy, so rather than being primarily concerned with whether your potential therapist is answering correctly or not, try to get a sense of this therapist's approach to determine if it's a good fit for you.

Would you please tell me about your general approach to therapy? This question can give you some insight into whether the therapist is oriented toward a focus on the whole person (psychodynamic, experiential, etc.) or on specific symptoms (cognitive-behavioral). There's no right or wrong answer, but it will tell you whether it's the type of therapy you're looking for.

Would you please tell me about your training, background and what license you have? This question is mainly to ensure you're working with someone who has the proper education and license to be conducting therapy. It's perfectly acceptable to work with pre-licensed therapists under supervision as long as they have an advanced degree and are working toward licensure.

Why did you become a therapist? While this question might make some therapists a little uncomfortable, it's perfectly fine to understand what someone's motivations were for entering the field. After all, you're going to be sharing deeply personal things with the person sitting in the room with you, and it can be good for the relationship for you to understand why someone is doing this type of work.

Are there any books that you'd recommend that I read to orient myself to our work? This type of question can give you a deeper insight into how your potential therapist views therapy. If you like to read, this can also provide you with resources outside of therapy sessions to deepen the work you're doing.

How long do you expect treatment to last? Again, there isn't a right or wrong answer to this question, but it does give you a sense whether or not this therapist's approach is in line with what you're looking for. Some therapies are open-ended and can go on for years, which is ok if that's what you want. Some are short-term and focused on specific symptoms or problems.

References

American Counseling Association (2014). 2014 ACA
Code of Ethics. Retrieved from
https://www.counseling.org/resources/aca-code-
of-ethics.pdf

Finn, J., & Barak, A. (2010). A descriptive study of e-
counsellor attitudes, ethics, and practice.
Counselling & Psychotherapy Research, 10(4),
268-277. doi:10.1080/14733140903380847

Li, L. P., Jaladin, R. M., & Abdullah, H. S. (2013).
Understanding the Two Sides of Online
Counseling and their Ethical and Legal
Ramifications. *Procedia - Social and Behavioral
Sciences, 103* (13th International Educational
Technology Conference), 1243-1251.
doi:10.1016/j.sbspro.2013.10.453

Oravec, J. A. (2000). Online counselling and the internet:
Perspectives for mental health care supervision

and education. *Journal of Mental Health*, *9*(2), 121-135. doi:10.1080/09638230050009122

Rummell, C. M., & Joyce, N. R. (2010). 'So wat do u want to wrk on 2day?': The Ethical Implications of Online Counseling. *Ethics & Behavior*, *20*(6), 482-496. doi:10.1080/10508422.2010.521450

Sperry, L. & Carlson, J. (2013). How master therapists work. New York, NY: Routledge.

Wampold BE. How important are the common factors in psychotherapy? An update. *World Psychiatry*. 2015;14(3):270–7. 10.1002/wps.20238

About the Author

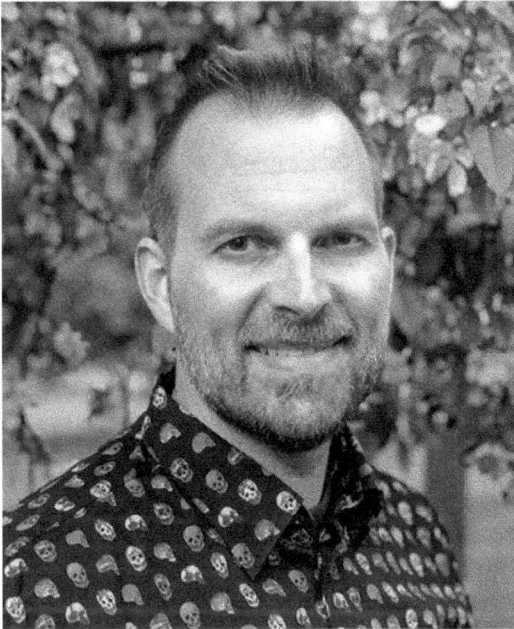

Ian Felton, MA, LPC, is a psychotherapist and mental health counselor in Minneapolis who holds a master's degree in Counseling & Psychological Services. He also has more than 20 years of experience writing software for organizations such as NASA and Mayo Clinic and is the author of The Coding Samurai: The Way of the

About the Author

Computer Warrior. *In addition to bass guitar, writing, and wildlife photography, his interests include Chinese language and facets of Chinese culture including philosophy, martial arts, and tea.*